Copyright © 2025 Christopher Welker
All rights reserved.

ISBN: 979-8-9933329-0-1
HUSHMARK Press

Printed by Amazon KDP

Acknowledgments

To the scientists, doctors, nurses, and medical staff who continue to show up — thank you.

For the research you do.
For the hours you work.
For the care you try to give, even when the system makes it difficult.

I know what it costs to keep doing this work.
I've seen the good it makes possible.

This book doesn't always speak kindly about the system.
But this page is for you.
Not as apology —
as gratitude.

You were there.
And I'm still here.

Thank you.

DIAGNOSIS

Blunt instruments
against my skin.

The pressure
within my mind.

Unbearable, raging
as my reality twists.

Searching for answers before rage
consumes me.

When will this
feeling end?

Arms bruised from IVs.
So many treatments.

Poisoning my body
Just to keep functioning.

Those are the choices
You have to make.

Eyes close
drifting off
in a hospital bed.

Incessant beeping.
Yelling down the hallway.

Exhausted.

Poked and prodded.
Endless testing.

You won't get better here.

Brain fractures
separated from
body.

Mind intact
as the body fails.

Pushing thru each day.
Before the body gives out.

Walking thru the door
straight to bed.

Pieces of the body
splinter from disease.

Body parts taken
to cure symptoms.

Replacement parts
for those removed.

How long will these last?
I'm left wondering.

Sticker and wires
attached in pattern.

Machine watching my pulse.

Automated machines
designed for alerting.

Wire falls off
nurses rush in.

I'm fine.

In my bed.
Tilted as my body fails.

Did I deserve this?
Is this a test?

Anger turns
to seething.

But it's no use.
There is only
one way
forward.

Night ruptured by pain.

Sleep taken from me.

Body fighting itself.

Will I get rest?

Hope drains.

From my mind.

From my body.

Fight to hang on.

Drift into sleep.

I rise bracing for
how my body feels.

What will the day bring?
Good?
Bad?
Or survival?

Everyday my body fights itself.

I'm just
the battlefield.

My face strained from tension.

People watching
silently.

As I move through days.

Reacting to signs
negatively.

While keeping everything together.

While this disease takes
everything
it can.

My body screams.
My mouth mute.

Who sees the struggle?

Who cares how much this disease takes.

Comfort doesn't come when you look fine.

It only comes when
you're broken.

The long loop of
chronic disease.

Never ending.

Feel better. Feel worse.

Doctors.

Canceled plans.

Who controls your life?

You? Disease?

Morphine hits my veins.

Buzz shift taking the edge from the pain.

Clouding my brain.

Relief brief.

Stomach cramps.

Trade one pain for another.

The trade off is swift.

Overhead lights bright.
Vision blurred.

Doctors talking.
Trying to make sense.

Severe.
Disease.

Acute treatment.

How did we get here?

Strangers. Glance in my direction.

As I'm called in.
Some familiar faces.

No one talks.
How sick am I?
Compared to others?

Why am I always the youngest one?

No one is with me.

I'm always at these
alone.

There is still trace amounts of blood.

My partner gasps.
I comfort them.

It's a good thing.

They look at me. Oddly?

I nod.

It used to be more.

TREATMENT

Tinge of
metal aftertaste.

After ingesting multiple antibiotics.

Medicine starts to
maintain day to day activities.

Small price for the
metal aftertaste

Diagnosis echoes inside.

The sad faces stop
looking at me.

They move on.

While I sit with
echoes,
reminders,
visages
of what once was.

Moving on but
forever changed.

Early doctor appointments.

Because they aren't late.

Can't keep asking for time off.

Guilt, shame.

I'll be in late is easier than
I need to leave for an appointment.

Especially when seeing
five   doctors
consistently.

Will they fire me?

Forming my life,
plans, relationships
based on how I feel.

People ask how I'm feeling.

I'm ok.
No one wants the
truth.

Because what will
they do with it?

I'm fine.

MRI.
CT Scan.
Blood Tests.

How many screenings
need to be done?

Before they know
what's wrong with me?

How many wait, prick, test
will I need?

We need to get
you the right
medicine.

This is working, I murmur.

You can't take
these
long term.

Why?

They are
bad for
you.

You'll adjust.
That's what those close say.

You'll figure it out.
What they always say.

You're tough.
That's what they say.

Compassion is only given.
Till I need to work harder.

Everyone forgets.
When their job is on the line.

The cost only grows.
Till the body fails.

Only compassion
when the body visibly breaks.

What's wrong
with you?

A flare.
When will you
be better?

I don't know.

I need you
to work on this project.

Ok.

Mom.

Dad.

I'm sick.

Pause.

How?

I don't know.

Is it treatable?

No.

Did you do this

to yourself?

What?

Do you have
a note?

Huh?
Why?

Proof that
you're sick?

You only have
so many
sick days.

I know.

I'll work extra.

I'm sorry.

How many pills?

How often do
I take them?

When is my
next appointment?

With who?

Can I have the
day off?

Yeah.

Just make you get your
work done.

Looking at the chart.
No words, just reading.

Paper wrinkles
underneath me.

Waiting.

Hands curled
against the edge
paper tearing.

How do you
feel?

Door opens.

Name called out.

I get up
and follow.

Wait for the
double zero.

I exhale.

Step on the scale.

Weight is announced.

Prednisone.
I whisper.

Following toward
the room.

Sit anywhere.

I watch my vitals.
Betraying me.

Prednisone.
60 mg.

Hands me a schedule.

Tapering over
weeks.

Rage.
Hunger.
Anger.

Breaking down
from the cost
to just function.

Then another cycle.

Prednisone.
60 mg.

Pharmacist
recognizes
me.

There is a problem.
Refill denied.

Why?

A shrug.

Ok.

Call your insurance
for help.

No more refills
there.

Refills only at
pharmacy
that we
own.

We'll try new medicine.
Hopefully, improve symptoms.

It's expensive.
How much?

Thousands.

Pharmacist scans
prescription.

Unfortunately, can't fill this.

I exhale slowly.

Call your
insurance
company.

I nod.

Phone rings.

Hello?

We need to reschedule
your visit?

When?
Two weeks.

I need more medicine
I'm almost out.

What's your pharmacy?

Next visit.

Overhearing the great
vacation the doctor had.

Two weeks ago.

New patient?

Fill out this paperwork
and hand it back
when done.

Clipboard in my lap.
Hunched over every paper.

Writing extra neat.

Financial responsible.
Me.

Emergency contact.
N/A.

Hand paperwork back.
Sitting down.

You forgot to sign
they call out.

In the waiting room.

Pharmaceutical rep
walks in.

Here to see the doctor.

They say and disappears
through the locked door.

In the exam room.

Waiting.

Let's try a new formulation
of your medicine.

It just came out.

Sitting on the
floor.

In our apartment.

While machine
I'm attached to beeps.

What's wrong with it?
I don't know.

I just have a number
for the company.

I call.
No answer.

Closing my eyes
while I'm cracking.

The beeping stops.

Laying in the hospital.

You need a
breathing treatment.

For what?

We saw something.

Saw what?

Something.

Who sent you?

The doctor.

Which doctor?

I look at the nurse.

They whisper
you can refuse it.

I don't want the treatment.

Nurse enters the room.

We have new medicines
to give you.

What?

Blood thinners.

I groan.

Those burn so bad.
I'll let you pick the place.

Ouch. The bee sting.

Don't rub it.

PERSISTENCE

Roll out of bed.

Looking at the clock.

How do I feel today?

Meh.

Wash up.

Reach for my pill box.

Out the door.

Body failing.

It's time they say.

I shake my head.

Not yet.

It's time they say.

Not yet.

Deeper into
sickness.

You don't
have a
choice.

When doctors
no longer give you.

Choice.

They move
with speed.

Wheeled into
so many exam rooms.

CT Scans.
MRIs.
Ultrasounds.

Some stat.
Some not.

I've lost count.

Rooms all look

the same.

But the hum is

familiar.

News Flash.

Most of these machines aren't maintained well.

Most people don't have enough of tests.

To worry.

How many tests?
Is enough to worry?

I've lost count.

How many
times a day
do you experience
symptoms?

I dunno.

Four?
Six?

I can only tell you
better or worse
than average.

I look at
my pills.

Becoming less compliant
day after day.

Are they making
a difference?

Does anything?

I get slower, sicker.

But still not compliant.

Fatigue.

I hate this
disease.

Why does it
still hurt?

When was your surgery?

Sixteen years ago.

Scar tissue.

Laying in recovery.

Stomach on fire.

Help it hurts.

Imagine it with
no pain meds. They whisper.

No it hurts.

On.

Fire.

Do you feel this?

I whimper Yes.

Oh.

Blacked out.

Coming to I hear.

Don't worry he can't
kill himself.

Patience stretching thin
after the fourth IV
prick.

I sigh.

Let's try
the other arm.

Ok.

I need the medicine.

I stare at IV
bags of chemicals.

Slowly dripping
into tubes.

Small bubbles.

Will it help?

We have to try it.

I don't feel well.

Nurse checks
all IV bags and
tubes.

It's probably
this one.

Holding bag #5
on the IV
stand.

I nod.

I bend
my arm.

Monitor blares
in response.

I straighten
my arm.

It stops.

I bend
my arm.

Monitor blares
in response.

I straighten
my arm.

It stops.

I bend
my arm.

...

Sitting in a chair.

Next to the doctor.
While they read
the screen.

I think…

Bracing.

It's time…

Shifting, gripping
the chair.

We might…

Sitting forward.

Need to…

Try…

Something else.

How long will
this surgery hold?

I keep asking
 myself.

Maybe   fifteen.
Maybe   twenty.
Years.

I keep
hoping
it will
last
longer.

Heading toward.

Another surgery.

Inconsistent intervals.

Appointments.
Medicines.

Take as close
if you miss a
dose.

Medicines never
formed
habit.

QD. (Once a day)

BID. (Twice a day)

TID. (Three times a day)

Every prescription
brings a
different schedule.

I finish
the infusion.

Arm wrapped with care.

Do you have your
next appointment?

Yes.

See you in 8 weeks.

Ok.

Pulling my sleeve down.

Walking out to work.

www.ingramcontent.com/pod-product-compliance
Lightning Source LLC
Chambersburg PA
CBHW042335150426
43194CB00005B/167